The Ultimate

How To Train For a 5K, 10K, Half-Marathon or Full Marathon

J. M. Parker

Copyright 2012

ISBN-13: 978-1478363347

ISBN-10: 1478363347

Disclaimer

This book is copyrighted with all rights reserved. No part of this book may be used in any form, physical or electronic, without express permission from the author.

The author does not assume any liability for the use or misuse of information contained herein. The information contained within this guide is for educational purposes and is offered as-is. The author does not assume any responsibility for the accuracy or misuse of any information contained herein.

While every attempt has been made to provide information that is both accurate and proven effective, the author and publisher make no guarantees that the information presented herein will benefit everyone in every situation. Everyone's situation is unique. The author assumes no liabilities for any use, misuse, injury or misconduct as a result of information within this book. As with all things that have to do with your body, if in doubt consult with your health care practitioner.

Table of Contents

Disclaimer 2
Table of Contents 1
About the Author 2
So You Wanna Run? 3
Why 26.2? 4
First things first… DIET! DIET DIET! 5
Bonus: Dining Out Tips 16
Hydrate! 18
Electrolytes 20
Stand up Straight! Stop Slouching! Head and Eyes to the Front! Proper Running Form 21
Choosing The Right Shoes 24
Gear up 27
Visualize 29
Anaerobic Fitness Versus Aerobic Fitness 32
Rate of Perceived Exertion 36
Strength Training-Don't Ignore It 37
Core Strength 38
Now Hit The Ground Running-Literally 40
The Master Plan! 42

Lower Body Exercise 49

Total Body Moves 56

More About Your Core 63

Interval Training 66

Common Running Injuries 69

Avoiding Burn Out 73

Crossing The Finish Line 75

Resource Section 76

About the Author

The author is a twelve year Army veteran who used to train soldiers to remain in compliance with Army height and weight standards in order to help them keep their careers. She has worked with many soldiers to complete the Army Birthday Annual Ten-Miler, and to get them down to a healthy height and weight. She is also certified to work with pregnant and post-partum women to safely maintain their fitness during pregnancy and to bounce back after child birth.

Post Army, the author still leads an active lifestyle and is pursuing a physical training certification and training for a local marathon.

So You Wanna Run?

Ok, then let's run. But it's not going to be easy and this no nonsense program is not for the faint of heart. If you want to run with us, you can't be a punk! Running a marathon is not for the weak bodied or for the fragile spirited.

The physical part of running is only a small portion of how far you can go. It's your mind that will carry you past the physical obstacles. You will feel pain during your training, but it's just weakness leaving the body. Don't cry. Just push through it and stop whining!

If you want to earn that 26.2 bumper sticker, this book will help you get it, but don't think you won't be pushed out of your comfort zone. Comfort is the thief of progress.

We don't want to rob you of your progress, so we'll make sure you are anything but comfortable. You may be in pain and you may be tired, but if you stick with it, you'll be glad you did. There's nothing quite like knowing you've accomplished a feat that makes you part of an elite group. It's not every day someone runs 26.2 miles.

So, if you're truly ready, grab your sneakers, your water bottle and this book to get started. Stay motivated, and stay disciplined. It's all worth it when you cross that finish line. Besides, no one likes a quitter.

Why 26.2?

As you may have gathered, anything over five miles is a pretty good haul, but why is a marathon so long? And why is it 26.2 miles, instead of 25 miles, or 30? Why don't marathons have the well defined distances of other races such as a 5k or 10k?

Legend has it that when the Greeks defeated a Persian naval invasion in 490 BC, a soldier named Pheidippides ran from the battlefield in Marathon, Greece, to Athens and delivered the news of the Greek victory. The distance between the cities was approximately 26.2 miles. The first marathon event in history commemorated this battle.

 Unfortunately, Pheidippides wasn't in the greatest shape. When he made it to Athens, he shouted "victory" then fell over and died. Lucky for you, we'll give you the tools you need get in top shape so that you'll cross the finish line alive and well, unlike poor Pheidippides. Too bad he didn't have this book back then.

First things first... DIET! DIET DIET!

This program is designed to help you complete a marathon. It's not a weight loss program, but if you do it right, weight loss can be a nice side effect.

You need to fuel your body to get through 26.2 miles. Don't be like Pheidippides. If you don't make it through the race, how are you going to brag about it later?

Right now is a great time to get all the junk out of your kitchen and start fresh with a clean, high protein diet. Get rid of the fatty cakes and get motivated!

No one is saying you have to give up everything you love for good but you do need to minimize it while you train. If you catch yourself craving a cookie, donut, potato chips or other items that you know aren't good for you, just say no. Go for a walk (or run), read a magazine, do a crossword puzzle. Do anything but give in. If distraction doesn't work, then go ahead and have a SMALL portion of what you're craving. Denying yourself could end up leading to a binge fest, so it's acceptable to give in to what you want, SOMETIMES.

Of course, you can't give into your cravings if the items aren't within your reach. So, open up your refrigerator and your cabinets and toss out anything containing simple carbohydrates, refined sugars, high sodium, and trans fats.

Now, if you want any unhealthy snacks, you'll have to go to the store and get them. Hopefully that will discourage you.

Get educated on how to read labels. Don't be misled by shiny, pretty labels that claim to be healthy. Some products masquerade as "sugar free" but contain other ingredients such as sucrose, high fructose corn syrup and xylitol. Those are all fancy words for sugar. If the sugar doesn't naturally occur in your food, it's best to leave it alone. Simple carbohydrates are foods made from grains, then bleached and sucked free of their nutritional value. Not all simple carbs are high calorie, but they all cause a high rise in your blood sugar, followed by steep drop, which is then followed by extreme hunger. Also, simple carbs that aren't burned off end up being stored as fat in your body. Excess fat will only slow you down on race day. Fatties don't make good runners, generally speaking.

To keep hunger pangs at pay, and keep your waistline in check, only buy carbohydrates made from whole grains, meaning complex carbohydrates. These carbs burn slowly and keep you feeling full longer. Beware the products that try to trick you with phrases like "multi-grain" or "100% wheat. Such phrases mean the products are not whole grain, but manufacturers want to trick you into thinking they are. Don't let them fool you! Think about it, just because something contains multiple grains doesn't mean those grains haven't been bleached and refined. If the word "whole" doesn't precede the word "grain," then just say "no."

Trans fats have been linked to health problems ranging from low energy to cancer. Most are found in your cooking oil. Fortunately, most foods are now made without trans fats, but check labels anyway. The Food and Drug Administration now requires companies to list the amount of trans fats found in their products. If a label shows ANY amount of trans-fats, your best bet is to pass it by.

Sodium doesn't pose many health risks for someone in their twenties and thirties, but it does increase your blood pressure, so if you have any sort of heart problems, you should limit your sodium intake to 2400 milligrams, if you're following a 2000 calorie diet. If your heart is healthy, sodium isn't much of a threat, but it can cause you to retain water and feel bloated, so limit the salty foods. Being bloated on race day is not a good feeling.

Now that you've cleared your kitchen of all the junk, it's time to stock up on the foods that will keep you going while you train, and during the race. Your diet should be made up of protein, fiber, calcium, whole grains and plenty of fruits and veggies.

Proteins: These are the building blocks of your muscles. You need muscles to carry you through the race. Remember, we don't like weakness, so get your protein and stay strong. Get lean protein from sources such as chicken, turkey, eggs, and lean beef. If you are not much of a meat eater, you can get protein from peanut butters, nuts, milk, cheese and tofu. There are also protein enriched whole grains on the market, but it's best to get it from foods that naturally have it. Scientists don't know why, but the body absorbs nutrients better when you eat foods that naturally contain them.

Fiber: Another source of long lasting energy, fiber also helps keep you going, so to speak. Fiber keeps your bowel movements regular. This is more important than you think. No one wants to run 26.2 mile while they're full of… impurities. It's very awkward. Try to incorporate fiber into every meal. You can find it naturally in items such as whole grains, beans, avocado, broccoli and carrots. Since you should be eating vegetables with lunch and dinner, and as your after lunch snack, you have plenty of opportunities to get your fiber fill.

Calcium: This is especially important if you're a woman. We aren't suggesting this nutrient simply for training for a marathon either. This is a long term necessity to ward of ailments such as osteoporosis. As you age, your bone density decreases, so get enough calcium now as a preemptive strike.

For marathon purposes, calcium is important because running can put a lot of impact on your joints and bones. Weak bones are counterproductive. We will show you how to reduce the impact and shock of hitting the pavement, but you still need strong bones to support you through the race. Like grains, check labels because many dairy products contain a high amount of refined sugars. Get calcium from sources such as low fat milk, cheese, yogurt, and fortified orange juice. An added bonus of calcium is that most dairy products also have protein. Keep your bones strong and you'll finish strong.

Whole grains: Remember the lasting energy we mentioned with fiber? Well, wholes grains can do it too. Buy whole grain breads, cereals and granola products. As always, check labels, because whole grain and sugar free aren't necessarily synonymous. This is especially true with cereal and granola. Refined sugars will give you a burst of energy, but when it wears off, you'll feel sluggish and tired. This isn't a good feeling while you run.

Fruits and veggies: Fruits and vegetables provide a wealth of benefits. Your momma didn't tell you to eat them for nothing! Well for this training, consider us your momma! They are packed with nutrients and antioxidants that boost your immune system and fight diseases such as cancer and heart disease. Every time you eat, half of your plate should contain produce. The more colorful your choices, the more health benefits you'll get from them. Try to eat everything from dark leafy greens to blueberries.

Below is a one week meal plan to get you started on the path to healthy eating, which will complement your active lifestyle. No fatty cakes on this menu folks! Clean and healthy is all we have here! If you want your milk and cookies, keep it moving, we can't accommodate that request!

Monday
Breakfast:
-Two hard-boiled eggs (you can eat the yolk)
-Smoothie containing 1 banana, 4 strawberries, 10 blackberries, a half a cup of Greek yogurt, either plain or vanilla, a few spinach leaves and ice. (don't worry about the spinach, you won't taste it, but you WILL reap the benefits of it.) Grind it all up and enjoy. Use honey or agave nectar to sweeten it. Also, you can use frozen fruit and skip the ice to save time.
-Granola bar (make sure it's low sugar, organic is best)
Lunch:
-Salad with baby spinach leaves or romaine lettuce, tomatoes, kidney beans, sunflower seeds, broccoli florets and grilled chicken strips.
-Use low fat dressing, or Balsamic vinegar and extra virgin olive oil. Feel free to add more veggies to this if you'd like
Dinner:
-Grilled fish (salmon, tilapia, halibut, tuna fish, etc)
-Steamed mixed vegetables
-Roasted red potatoes with rosemary and cherry tomatoes.

Tuesday
Breakfast
-Whole grain bagel with one Laughing Cow or Weight Watchers cheese wedge.
-One half grapefruit, sweetened with Stevia

-3 Strips of turkey bacon

Lunch

-Turkey breast sandwich on whole grain bread with lettuce and tomatoes

-Garden salad or minestrone soup

-Low-fat yogurt

Dinner

-Grilled chicken breast

-Steamed asparagus

-Brown Rice

Wednesday

Breakfast

-Greek yogurt with honey and granola

-Skim milk latte

-Cup of sliced melon

Lunch

-Veggie burger on whole grain bun with lettuce and tomatoes

-Steamed mixed veggies

-Frozen baked French fries

Dinner

-3 oz lean steak

-Summer squash

-Baked Sweet potato

Thursday

Breakfast

-Whole grain cereal (Kashi and Special K make excellent ones) with skim milk
-Orange slices
-Whole grain toast with peanut butter
Lunch
-Whole grain pita with chicken breast, plain Greek yogurt, tomatoes and olives
-Garden salad
Dinner
-Whole grain spaghetti with marinara sauce and ground turkey meat balls
-Bruschetta with whole grain bread

Friday
Breakfast
-Oatmeal with walnuts, milk honey and cinnamon
-Apple
Lunch
-Tomato soup with Triscuits
-Baby carrots and fat free cream cheese
Dinner
-Chicken fajitas with fat free sour cream on whole grain tortillas

Saturday
Breakfast
-Egg White omelets with low fat cheddar cheese, diced green peppers, tomatoes and low-fat ham
-Bowl of mixed fruits

Lunch

-Grilled Chicken salad

- Your choice of low fat soup

Dinner

-Roasted pork loin

-Boiled artichokes

-Roasted russet potatoes

Sunday

Breakfast

-Whole grain toaster waffles with sugar free syrup

-Strawberry and blackberry parfait

Lunch

-Spaghetti squash with marinara sauce

-Grilled chicken breast

Dinner

-Grilled fish

-Steamed broccoli

-Baked russet potatoes

Snacks

-Nuts, especially almonds, cashews and walnuts

-Yogurt

-Low sugar granola

-Skim milk lattes

-Veggies and hummus

-Vegetable chips
-Dried fruit (check sugar content)
-Your choice of fruits and veggies

Dessert Options
-Strawberry shortcake, but use fat free angel food cake instead of short cake and use fat free whipped topping
-Fruit and yogurt parfait
-Frozen yogurt milk shakes
-Chocolate covered strawberries (in moderation)

The meal plan we've provided is just a small sample of the possibilities for a healthy diet. You have plenty of non-junk, not fatty cake options available to you, so use them.

There are countless foods that are good for you and countless ways to prepare them. There's no excuse for not eating right, especially if you are active. We'd say running a marathon is pretty active. After about three weeks of eating the right way, your cravings for the bad stuff will likely disappear, or at least visit you less frequently.

Whatever you do while training, do NOT starve yourself. Runners need more calories than those who lead a sedentary lifestyle. Eat smaller meals every 3-4 hours to keep your blood sugar stable and keep your energy up. Make sure you enjoy what you're eating, because if you're unhappy with the food you're consuming, you'll revert back to the junk food that slows you down. Variety is key here too. Boredom ALWAYS kills your best efforts to eat right. Don't get bored. Keep your taste buds guessing and happy.

Losing weight shouldn't be your only motivation for completing a marathon. If weight loss is your only goal, you're not very likely to finish. However, if you'd like to lose weight while you train for other reasons (glory, charity, fun, bragging rights) all you need to do is work out and follow our tips. There is no magic pill to get you to your goal weight overnight. Stay away from fad diets and elimination diets. Just consume fewer calories than you expend and you'll be fine. Put that donut down and pay attention! We are trying to help!

If you don't fuel yourself properly, you may end up passing out before you can make it halfway through the race. Don't be that guy. Be the guy that follows our advice and makes this event a success.

Bonus: Dining Out Tips

Now that you're armed with the knowledge you need to keep your diet in check, we have some advice to give you on dining out. The most important thing: PLAN AHEAD. If you intend to dine at a chain restaurant, look up the nutrition information before you go, and choose your meal before you get there. Some restaurants have nutritional information on the menu, so you can use that as a guide if you prefer.

If you can't find the information online, then look up the nutrition facts for the types of food served at the restaurant you plan on visiting. Also, ask the waiter how the food is prepared. As much as we've talked about whole grains, there might be an exception to that rule when dining out. Often times, Hibachi style restaurants prepare their brown rice with butter, but steam their white rice. In instances such as these, it's better to get the lower calorie simple carbohydrates than the calorie loaded complex ones.

It all comes down to doing your research and preparing ahead of time. It's also about eating right the day you plan on dining out. Don't make the mistake of starving yourself to save calories and eat like it's your last meal when you get to the restaurant. Just scale back on the calories in your foods throughout the day. Don't eliminate any meals, although skipping a snack won't hurt. Still holding that donut? LET IT GO!!

If you are meeting friends for cocktails, tread lightly. Alcohol has more calories than you think. It's hard to imagine, since most alcoholic beverages don't include nutrition labels on the bottle. Some lighter options include mojitos, margaritas and martinis. Avoid drinks that add sugary extras such as pina colada, rum and coke, and daiquiris. And know your limit! Don't get trashed and render yourself unable to train the following day! If you know you're a lightweight, drink accordingly! Put down that last tequila shot!

Hydrate!

Now that you've been schooled on how to properly fuel yourself for a marathon, it's time to teach you how to hydrate. Hydration is essential during training, and while you run.

Lack of hydration has literally been the death of many athletes. We definitely don't want you to die before, or after crossing the finish line, so make sure you're getting plenty of water. Don't be like Pheidippides! We'd be willing to bet that if he had been properly hydrated he wouldn't have keeled over like that.

Luckily, the old rule of chugging eight glasses of water every day no longer applies. Many foods can provide plenty of water. Try filling up on foods like watermelon, grapes, strawberries, and tomatoes. Water is also found in unexpected sources such as oatmeal, which is 84% water and lean yogurt, which is 79% water.

You can't give water up completely and get all of it from your food, but you can scale back and perhaps avoid the dreaded side cramp during your runs.

Don't take salt pills in an attempt to retain water. Many years ago, soldiers had to take salt pills because of the large amounts of water they were losing in combat. Some still follow this antiquated practice. The problem is that you NEED to sweat. Sweat is your body's way of cooling down. Cooling down prevents heat injuries such as heat cramps, heat exhaustion and heat stroke. Simply replace the water you lose by drinking water or eating foods with high water content. The salt in your foods should be sufficient to prevent you from losing too much water.

Don't wait until you are thirsty to hydrate. Thirst is actually an early sign of dehydration. If you are thirsty, you've waited too long.

Another sign of dehydration: your pee. No one wants to look in the toilet after using it, but it's a great way to know if you're properly hydrated. Your urine should be light or clear. Dark urine is an indicator of dehydration so unfortunately, you need to monitor your pee. Who cares if it's nasty?! Just look!

Electrolytes

If you thought you could drink some water and be on your way, you thought wrong. Everyone's body has electrically charged ions in them called electrolytes. Their purpose in life is to help your cells maintain the voltage in your cell membranes and to carry electrical impulses, such as muscle contractions, throughout your body.

To maintain the balance of electrolytes in your body, drink a sports drink such as Gatorade or Power Aid after an intense work out. They replenish much of what is lost during a workout. Don't replace your water with sports drinks though. They are full of refined sugar, which is your enemy most of the time. Just one a day after a workout will suffice.

Stand up Straight! Stop Slouching! Head and Eyes to the Front! Proper Running Form

An often ignored factor that may determine the outcome of your race is your form. Improper form can cause unnecessary strain and impact on your joints, back, hips and legs. Over time, this impact can cause longer term problems such as stress fractures and tendonitis, neither of which make good running partners. Besides, does anyone really want to look like a goofball while they run? Self consciousness slows you down.

From your head to your feet, and everywhere in between, your body needs to be properly aligned to lessen the risk of injury and to lessen the pain your muscles and joints. You'll also run faster if you run properly. So, stand up straight! Stop Slouching! Head and eyes to the front!

Keep reading to learn more.

Posture

First off, look straight ahead, about five to ten feet in front of you. Don't look at the ground, or at the sky. Keep your head high, aligned with your spine and centered between your shoulders. Stand with your shoulders pulled back, as though you are trying to make your shoulder blades touch, and make sure your arms are at a ninety degree angle to the running surface.

Make sure your feet are pointed ahead, and not turned in or out. They should be pointed in the direction that you are running, which is forward.

Hands and Arms

Now, pay attention to your arms and hands. You'd be surprised at how fast you can become fatigued by clenching your fists or holding your arms up too high. Keep your hands cupped as though you're holding an egg in each one. Your elbows should be bent at 90 degrees. As you pump your arms, your elbows should be between your waistline and chest. The faster you pump your arms, the more leg turnover you can manage. More leg turnover means a faster run time, which means more glory at the finish line.

Breathing

Breathe deeply, from your diaphragm. To practice this skill, lie down on your back, and put a book or other flat object on your stomach. Inhale slowly and observe the book rising, then exhale to see it falling. Who cares if you feel silly doing it? It'll help you, so grab your book and do what we tell you!

If you're not embarrassed, call cadence. If you are embarrassed, call it in your brain. Running to a rhythm helps you control your breathing better, and also helps distract you so that the time passes much faster. We know it hurts! Don't cry. Sing!

Striking the Ground (Foot strike)

Your foot should hit the ground from the center of your foot and you should roll through the front of your feet, the padded portion next to your toes. If your foot strikes with the front first, it will cause fatigue in your calves and pain in your shins. Hitting the ground with your heels puts more impact on your hips, and slows you down.

Try not to pound the pavement. Be light on your feet to reduce the shock on your joints that we keep mentioning. We're talking about it for a reason people!

Hit the Hills

During an uphill interval, lift your knees up, shorten your stride and pump your arms faster. Lean into the hill to help pull you up.

When running downhill, lower your arms, hold your body at the same angle as the hill and try to land so that the front of your foot hits first. Don't lean from your waist. Lean from your ankles.

While we're on the topic of hills, make sure you incorporate them in your training program. Hill runs build lower body strength and help to improve your speed.

Choosing The Right Shoes

Don't just grab a pair of shoes that fits and hit the road. It's much more involved than that. The right pair of shoes is critical to your success in the race, and to preventing injuries. You need shoes that support your arches and ankles, that fit properly and that absorb shock well, to minimize the impact on your joints. See, there it is again… impact on your joints. It's only because we care. We want training to hurt you, but not in a bad way.

You don't need to be an expert in sports medicine or podiatry (and we're assuming you're not) to find the right shoes. You just need a foot specialty store. Most major athletic stores such as FootLocker have a digital posture and arch analysis machine. Their employees should be trained on the machines and on advising customers on the best shoes for their foot type.

The salesperson should measure your foot to determine your true shoe size. Your shoes should be a half or full size bigger than your regular shoe size, to accommodate the swelling that occurs when you run. If your shoes don't have adequate space for your toes, you could end up with blisters or nasty black toenails.

The salesperson will determine if you have high arches, low arches, fallen arches or flat feet. He or she will then observe you running and decide if your feet turn inward (pronated) or if they turn outward (supinated).

Let the salesperson know things such as how often you run, the fact that you're training for a marathon, what surface you run on and what type of running you do. Inform them of any injuries in your lower extremities, such as sprains, fractures or shin splints. You'll want a shoe with some extra support if this describes you.

With this information the sales person can recommend a pair of shoes for you. Don't try them on and walk a few steps. RUN in them before you decide. You'll be running in them while you train, and you'll be running in them on the day of the marathon, so walking in them now will do you no good. Shoes that work for you when you walk may not work as well when you run.

After you purchase your shoes, give them a one week trial. If after a week you develop blisters or pain, take the shoes back. Most stores have return policies that allow you to return shoes even after you've worn them.

Once you have the perfect pair of shoes, see if you can find them at a discounted rate online or in outlet stores. You don't have to go back to the same store each time you need a new pair of shoes. Replace your running shoes every 300-400 miles.

If you were a runner before you began this program, take your current running shoes with you to the store. The salesperson will ascertain quite a bit about your running style by the wear on your soles.

Make sure you are standing up when your feet are measured, as the measurement will be more accurate. After all, it's not like you will be sitting down while you run.

Bring your insoles or orthotics to try your shoes on. If you have them, you'll need to know that your shoes are roomy enough for them.

Don't worry about what the shoes look like. Style isn't as important here as what's best for your body. Ugly shoes that don't cause injury are better than cute ones that do. It's a marathon princess, not a fashion show!

Gear up

As important as your shoes is the rest of your outfit. Buy clothes made for running. We know this sounds obvious, but if you've ever tried to run a long distance in biker shorts you know why we're bringing this up. Talk about awkward!

Although we want some aspects of your training to be uncomfortable for you, we don't want to slow you down by not properly gearing up. Invest in a few pair of moisture wicking jogging pants, and tops that fit close to your body. You don't want loose clothing getting in your way while you run and you don't want to be bogged down with sweaty clothing. Once again, go for practicality over fashion. If you're that worried about what you're wearing, audition for a modeling gig and leave marathons alone.

If you're a female you'll need a good sports bra too. Even if you're not exactly endowed in that region, you'll want the support there. You can still feel pain there if you're not "held up," so to speak.

You probably don't need to carry a water bottle with you, because most long distance races have water and sports drinks stops along the way, usually every two miles or so. If you'd rather carry your own, get one with a lanyard so you can slip your hand through it. That way, if you accidentally let go, the bottle won't go rolling away from you in the opposite direction of where you're going. Another idea for carrying water around during the race is to invest in a camel back. If you plan on that, make sure you train with your camelback too, so that on race day you're used to running with it.

Your socks matter too. Don't wear socks so thick that they compromise the fit of your shoes and don't wear ones so thin that you get blisters. Typically a cotton and nylon blend with a little bit of cushioning work best.

Make sure everything you buy fits well. You don't want to waste time pulling your pants up, pulling your shirt down, or yanking your pants out of your nether-regions while you run. Trust us; it's not a good time!

Visualize

It may sound New Age to you, but you have to picture yourself being successful in this race in order to really be successful. If you go into it assuming you won't do well, you've created a self-fulfilling prophecy. So basically, you'll suck. The right mindset will take you very far in this event, and in life, so adopt that mind set now for long term success.

At some point during the race, you are going to want to quit. When your body wants to quit you'll have to rely on your mind to do the rest. So, even though you may think we sound like modern day hippies, take our advice and visualize.

No one says you have to light candles and meditate, but you do need to focus on the task at hand with a positive, optimistic attitude.

Some methods for keeping you focused and motivated follow:

-On days you want to skip a workout, tell yourself you'll workout for three minutes. Typically, it takes three minutes for those feel good endorphins to kick in and you'll want to keep going. Don't complain. Anyone can manage three minutes.

-Don't focus on how fast or slow others are running. Comparing yourself to other runners can get discouraging if they are all faster than you. Just worry about achieving your personal best. The last person to finish is still someone who can run 26.2 miles. How many people do you know who can do that?

-Picture yourself crossing the finish line every day. Imagine it while you train and it will become a reality on race day.

-Put "26.2" on sticky notes and place them where you're sure to see them; on the refrigerator, on the bathroom mirror, on your television, etc. Every time you see it you'll be reminded of the end result and you'll be pushed to keep going.

-Put 120% percent into everything you do. Not in the literal physical term (you should typically exercise at 90% of your max effort), but in general, try your hardest, and then try harder than that. In doing so, you'll still perform at 100% on the days you're feeling less than stellar. You'll only get from this program what you put into it, so put in as much as you can, and them some!

The more you focus, the easier it will be to get through your workouts and to get through the race itself. Most runners will tell you that running is almost as much mental as it is physical. When your body starts to protest and you feel like quitting, you'll need a strong mind and will power to keep you going and push past the pain.

We don't mean push past pain that might be indicative of an injury of course, but push past the discomfort. Remember, comfort is the thief of progress!

Anaerobic Fitness Versus Aerobic Fitness

Both forms of fitness are important to your overall health and you have to incorporate both while you train in order to maximize your performance.

Aerobic exercise refers to moderate paced, long lasting workouts such as distance runs, step classes, hikes and other workouts of that nature. The term aerobic literally means "with oxygen." When your heart rate is in the aerobic zone, your muscles are getting enough oxygen to sustain the energy needed to continue working out. Aerobic exercise has been linked to many health benefits including:

-Decreased risk of diabetes

-Weight loss

-Decreased risk of heart disease

-Decreased risk of certain cancers

-Increased endurance

-Improved Immune system

-Higher levels of good cholesterol and lower levels of bad

-Improvements in blood circulation and cardiovascular systems

-Decreased risk of stroke

If aerobic means "with oxygen" then anaerobic means, you guessed it, "without oxygen." Of course, you can't do ANYTHING without oxygen, let alone run 26.2 miles, but when the intensity of your workouts are so high that you don't get your energy from oxygen, your body starts using glycogen, which comes from carbohydrates. Anaerobic exercise includes weight training and High Intensity Interval Training (HIIT).

One of the best things about anaerobic exercise is that your body continues to torch calories even after you've stopped working out. It also provides the same benefits as aerobic training along with increased muscle mass and improved speed.

Most workouts will not be exclusively anaerobic, as your anaerobic system doesn't kick in until your aerobic system can no longer provide you with enough energy to keep going.

The chart below, known as the Fox and Haskell formula will help you determine which zone you are working out in. If you have ever used a cardio machine in the gym, you've probably seen this chart before. The maximum heart is different for everyone, and the chart is not definitive, but it's a good guideline to use in determining if you need to go harder or slow down. Be alert and look for signs from your body that could indicate overexertion. If you feel weak or lightheaded, don't worry about your heart rate. Stop, drink some water and regroup.

EXERCISE ZONES

BEATS PER MINUTE		AGE									
		20	25	30	35	40	45	50	55	65	70
	100%	200	195	190	185	180	175	170	165	155	150
		VO2 Max (Maximum effort)									
	90%	180	176	171	167	162	158	153	149	140	135
		Anaerobic (Hardcore training)									
	80%	160	156	152	148	144	140	136	132	124	120
		Aerobic (Cardio training / Endurance)									
	70%	140	137	133	130	126	123	119	116	109	105
		Weight control (Fitness / Fat burn)									
	60%	120	117	114	111	108	105	102	99	93	90
		Moderate activity (Maintenance / Warm up)									
	50%	100	98	95	93	90	88	85	83	78	75

As indicated, the 70% zone is considered the weight control zone. Anything in this zone and beyond will torch calories very efficiently and build your stamina.

To obtain your heart rate, simply place your fingers on a pulse point, and count your heartbeats for 15 seconds. Then take that number and multiply by four and you'll know your beats per minute. Or you can purchase a pedometer or watch with a heart rate monitor on it.

Rate of Perceived Exertion

Many people have issues with the Fox and Haskell formula because it doesn't take into account individual fitness levels. If you would rather not bother with counting your heart rate or attempting to determine out what's right for your personal fitness level, you'll be better off using the Rate of Perceived Exertion formula. Basically, your RPE is how hard your workout feels, on a scale of 1-10. The "talk test" is used to determine what number you use. The harder it is for you to talk, the more energy you're expending. Use the chart below to find your RPE.

RATE OF PERCIEVED EXERTION (RPE)		
SCALE	TALK TEST	% OF MAX HEART RATE
1-3	Talking in full sentences is easy. Requires almost no effort.	40-50%
4-5	You can still talk, but it's somewhat harder	50-60%
6-7	You can breath, but it's a challenge. Talking is hard and you'd rather not	60-70%
8-9	Breathing is difficult and holding a conversation is next to impossible	70-80%
10	You can't, and shouldn't sustain this level more than few seconds. You're gasping for air to speak.	90%

Strength Training-Don't Ignore It

It's easy to believe that in order to be prepared for a marathon that all you have to do is run, run and run some more.

If only that were true. While running is of course an integral aspect of your training, you can't ignore your muscular strength and endurance. The stronger your body is, the better able it is to carry you through the race.

Your muscles are what hold you up and support your body, so don't neglect them. Build muscle mass by weight training, and other resistance training. If you're a female and worried about adding too much bulk to your frame, don't be. Just lift lighter weights and perform more repetitions, or do exercises that use your body weight as resistance.

Incorporate strength training at least two days out of the week. Use one day to work out your lower body, and another to do total body exercises. Since your lower body will be doing most of the work while you run, it's highly important to keep it in excellent repair. Just because you're running doesn't mean you're building as much strength in your legs as you could be. Build them up more by doing squats, lunges and hill runs.

Core Strength

Here's another area of the body that often gets overlooked when training for a long distance race. Ignoring your core is a huge mistake. A weak core makes you a weak runner. We don't tolerate weakness, so get your core right.

Your core is more than just that coveted six pack in your abdominal area. Your core consists of a large group of muscles that run the entire length of your torso. A strong core reduces back pain, and improves your overall athletic performance. They are also the muscles that make standing up and walking possible. (You thought it was your legs didn't you?). The core is basically your body's internal girdle. A strong core allows for stronger movements.

One of the most common ways to improve core strength is by planking, where you hold your body in the push up position for a given amount of time. Planks are great, but don't stop there. Do exercises that put you off balance, or that use your upper and lower abs at the same time to really work those muscles. Try lifting weights on a Bosu ball, or do push-ups with your hands balancing you on a medicine ball. What's great about core exercises is that most of them target more than one muscle group at a time, giving you more work out in less time.

Your core should be worked out every day, no matter what other muscle groups are being worked. We realize it's difficult. Don't cry. Just do what we say.

Incorporate a fifteen minute core routine at the beginning or end of each of your workouts and not only will you end up with washboard abs, but you'll improve your balance and posture. Remember, don't ignore the core.

Now Hit The Ground Running-Literally

Now that we've covered the basics we can get into the main topic of this book: RUNNING! In this chapter we'll discuss the program we've developed for you to prepare for a 5k, 10k, half marathon and the Granddaddy of them all, the MARATHON!

This guide is for beginners, or veterans who have fallen off the wagon for awhile. We'll get you prepared for this monumental event by starting small, with a 5K, and working up to that 26.2 bumper sticker.

This is a 32 week program that can be adjusted to meet your individual fitness abilities. We start Week 1 with a nice and easy one mile run. If this is too easy for you, start in Week 2, or beyond. A half a mile is added each week until you've reached marathon distance.

Now, why some races are measured in kilometers and some in miles is a mystery to us. Perhaps it's because America is the only country that uses the standard system of measure, while the rest of the world uses the metric system. Whatever the reason, you can determine your miles using this simple formula: Multiply kilometers by 6.2 and drop the last number. For example, a 10k would be six miles, since 10 times 6.2 is 62. If you just want a ballpark figure, don't include the .2. Just multiply by six and drop the last number.

Since basic math might be hard for you, and many others, we took the liberty of creating the chart below to save you the time and headache of multiplication. You're welcome.

KM	MILES
1	0.62
10	6.21
20	12.43
30	18.64
40	24.85
50	31.07
60	37.28
70	43.5
80	49.71
90	55.62
100	62.14

The Master Plan!

What follows is the plan we've come up with to get you marathon ready! At a glance it may look monotonous, but we have a plan for that too. When you see "lower body" workout in your plan, you can choose from any of the lower body plans that we've included. The same thing applies to the total body workout.

Boredom is a motivation killer, so we've covered that. With our plan, you might be in pain, but you won't be bored.

Don't be intimidated by how many weeks this plan is, (intimidation is just a fancy word for scared and fear is a form of weakness) or by the distances you'll end up running. If you stick with it, running will become natural to you after a few weeks. The pages that follow offer ideas on workouts for your lower body, total body and core and runs. Mix and match the exercises as you please. Keeping your muscles guessing prevents you from hitting a plateau. If you don't find any of our ideas interesting, then get online, or get some fitness magazines. Either way, stay active and stay strong.

5 K Training
(4 Weeks)

Week 1

Mon	Tue	Wed	Thur	Fri
Run 1 Mile	Lower Body	Interval Tng 1 Mile	Total body/core	1.5 Miles

Week 2

Mon	Tue	Wed	Thur	Fri
Run 1.5 Miles	Lower body	Interval 1.5 Miles	Total body/core	2 Miles

Week 3

Mon	Tue	Wed	Thur	Fri
Run 2 Miles	Lower Body	Interval for 2 miles	Total Body/Core	2.5 Miles

Week 4

Mon	Tue	Wed	Thur	Fri
Run 2.5 Miles	Lower Body	Interval for 2 miles	Total Body/Core	3 Miles

10 K
(10 Weeks)

Week 1

Mon	Tue	Wed	Thur	Fri
Run 1 Mile	Lower Body	Interval Tng 1 Mile	Total body/core	1.5 Miles

Week 2

Mon	Tue	Wed	Thur	Fri
Run 1.5 Miles	Lower body	Interval 1.5 Miles	Total body/core	2 Miles

Week 3

Mon	Tue	Wed	Thur	Fri
Run 2 Miles	Lower Body	Interval for 2 miles	Total Body/Core	2.5 Miles

Week 4

Mon	Tue	Wed	Thur	Fri
Run 2.5 Miles	Lower Body	Interval for 2 miles	Total Body/Core	3 Miles

Week 5

Mon	Tue	Wed	Thur	Fri
Run 3 Miles	Lower Body	Interval for 2 miles	Total Body/Core	Run 3.5 Miles

Week 6

Mon	Tue	Wed	Thur	Fri

	Mon	Tue	Wed	Thur	Fri
	Run 3.5 Miles	Lower Body	Interval for 2 Miles	Total Body/Core	Run 4 Miles

Week 7

Mon	Tue	Wed	Thur	Fri
Run 4 Miles	Lower Body	Interval for 2 Miles	Total Body/Core	Run 4.5 Miles

Week 8

Mon	Tue	Wed	Thur	Fri
Run 4.5 Miles	Lower Body	Interval for 2 mIles	Total Body/core	Run 5 Miles

Week 9

Mon	Tue	Wed	Thur	Fri
Run 5 Miles	Lower Body	Interval for 2 Miles	Total Body/Core	Run 5.5 Miles

Week 10

Mon	Tue	Wed	Thur	Fri
Run 5.5 Miles	Lower Body	Interval for 2 miles	Total Body/Core	Run 6 miles

Half Marathon (18 Weeks)

Week 1

Mon	Tue	Wed	Thur	Fri
Run 1 Mile	Lower Body	Interval Tng 1 Mile	Total body/core	1.5 Miles

Week 2

Mon	Tue	Wed	Thur	Fri
Run 1.5 Miles	Lower body	Interval 1.5 Miles	Total body/core	2 Miles

Week 3

Mon	Tue	Wed	Thur	Fri
Run 2 Miles	Lower Body	Interval for 2 miles	Total Body/Core	2.5 Miles

Week 4

Mon	Tue	Wed	Thur	Fri
Run 2.5 Miles	Lower Body	Interval for 2 miles	Total Body/Core	3 Miles

Week 5

Mon	Tue	Wed	Thur	Fri
Run 3 Miles	Lower Body	Interval for 2 miles	Total Body/Core	Run 3.5 Miles

Week 6

Mon	Tue	Wed	Thur	Fri
Run 3.5 Miles	Lower Body	Interval for 2 Miles	Total Body/Core	Run 4 Miles

Week 7

Mon	Tue	Wed	Thur	Fri
Run 4 Miles	Lower Body	Interval for 2 Miles	Total Body/Core	Run 4.5 Miles

Week 8

Mon	Tue	Wed	Thur	Fri
Run 4.5 Miles	Lower Body	Interval for 2 mIles	Total Body/core	Run 5 Miles

Week 9

Mon	Tue	Wed	Thur	Fri
Run 5 Miles	Lower Body	Interval for 2 Miles	Total Body/Core	Run 5.5 Miles

Week 10

Mon	Tue	Wed	Thur	Fri
Run 5.5 Miles	Lower Body	Interval for 2 miles	Total Body/Core	Run 6 miles

Week 11

Mon	Tue	Wed	Thur	Fri
Run 6 Miles	Lower Body	3 Mile Interval	total Body/core	Run 6.5 Miles

Week 12

Mon	Tue	Wed	Thur	Fri
Run 7 Miles	Lower Body	3 Mile Interval	total body/core	Run 7.5 Miles

Week 13

Mon	Tue	Wed	Thur	Fri
Run 8 Miles	Lower Body	3 Mile Interval	total body/core	Run 8.5 Miles

Week 14

Mon	Tue	Wed	Thur	Fri
Run 9 Miles	Lower Body	3 Mile Interval	Total Body/Core	Run 9.5 Miles

Week 15

Mon	Tue	Wed	Thur	Fri
Run 10 Miles	Lower Body	3 Mile Interval	Total Body/Core	Run 10.5 miles

Week 16

Mon	Tue	Wed	Thur	Fri
Run 11 Miles	Lower Body	3 Mile Interval	Total Body/Core	Run 11.5Miles

Week 17

Mon	Tue	Wed	Thur	Fri
Run 12 Miles	Lower Body	3 Mile Interval	Total Body/Core	Run 12.5 Miles

Week 18

Mon	Tue	Wed	Thur	Fri
Run 13 Miles	Lower Body	3 Mile Interval	Total Body/Core	Run 13.5 Miles

**Marathon
(32 Weeks)**

Week 1

Mon	Tue	Wed	Thur	Fri
Run 1 Mile	Lower Body	1 Mile Interval	Total body/core	1.5 Miles

Week 2

Mon	Tue	Wed	Thur	Fri
Run 1.5 Miles	Lower body	Interval 1.5 Miles	Total body/core	2 Miles

Week 3

Mon	Tue	Wed	Thur	Fri
Run 2 Miles	Lower Body	Interval for 2 miles	Total Body/Core	2.5 Miles

Week 4

Mon	Tue	Wed	Thur	Fri
Run 2.5 Miles	Lower Body	Interval for 2 miles	Total Body/Core	3 Miles

Week 5

Mon	Tue	Wed	Thur	Fri
Run 3 Miles	Lower Body	Interval for 2 miles	Total Body/Core	Run 3.5 Miles

Week 6

Mon	Tue	Wed	Thur	Fri
Run 3.5 Miles	Lower Body	Interval for 2 Miles	Total Body/Core	Run 4 Miles

Week 7

Mon	Tue	Wed	Thur	Fri
Run 4 Miles	Lower Body	Interval for 2 Miles	Total Body/Core	Run 4.5 Miles

Week 8

Mon	Tue	Wed	Thur	Fri
Run 4.5 Miles	Lower Body	Interval for 2 mIles	Total Body/core	Run 5 Miles

Week 9

Mon	Tue	Wed	Thur	Fri
Run 5 Miles	Lower Body	Interval for 2 Miles	Total Body/Core	Run 5.5 Miles

Week 10

Mon	Tue	Wed	Thur	Fri
Run 5.5 Miles	Lower Body	Interval for 2 miles	Total Body/Core	Run 6 miles

Week 11

Mon	Tue	Wed	Thur	Fri

Run 6 Miles	Lower Body	3 Mile Interval	total Body/core	Run 6.5 Miles

Week 12
Mon	Tue	Wed	Thur	Fri
Run 7 Miles	Lower Body	3 Mile Interval	total body/core	Run 7.5 Miles

Week 13
Mon	Tue	Wed	Thur	Fri
Run 8 Miles	Lower Body	3 Mile Interval	total body/core	Run 8.5 Miles

Week 14
Mon	Tue	Wed	Thur	Fri
Run 9 Miles	Lower Body	3 Mile Interval	Total Body/Core	Run 9.5 Miles

Week 15
Mon	Tue	Wed	Thur	Fri
Run 10 Miles	Lower Body	3 Mile Interval	Total Body/Core	Run 10.5 miles

Week 16
Mon	Tue	Wed	Thur	Fri
Run 11 Miles	Lower Body	3 Mile Interval	Total Body/Core	Run 11.5Miles

Week 17
Mon	Tue	Wed	Thur	Fri
Run 12 Miles	Lower Body	3 Mile Interval	Total Body/Core	Run 12.5 Miles

Week 18
Mon	Tue	Wed	Thur	Fri
Run 13 Miles	Lower Body	3 Mile Interval	Total Body/Core	Run 13.5 Miles

Week 19
Mon	Tue	Wed	Thur	Fri
Run 14 Miles	Lower Body	3 Mile Interval	Total Body/Core	Run 14.5 Miles

Week 20
Mon	Tue	Wed	Thur	Fri
Run 15 Miles	Lower Body	3 Mile Interval	Total Body/Core	Run 15.5 Miles

Week 21
Mon	Tue	Wed	Thur	Fri
Run 16 Miles	Lower Body	3 Mile Interval	Total Body/Core	Run 16.5 Miles

Week 22
Mon	Tue	Wed	Thur	Fri
Run 17 Miles	Lower Body	3 Mile Interval	Total Body/Core	Run 17.5 Miles

Week 23
Mon	Tue	Wed	Thur	Fri
18 Run 18 Miles	Lower Body	3 Mile Interval	Total Body/Core	Run 18.5 Miles

Week 24
Mon	Tue	Wed	Thur	Fri
Run 19 Miles	Lower Body	3 Mile Interval	Total Body/Core	Run 20 Miles

Week 25
Mon	Tue	Wed	Thur	Fri
Run 20 Miles	Lower Body	3 Mile Interval	Total Body/Core	Run 21 Miles

Week 26
Mon	Tue	Wed	Thur	Fri
Run 21 Miles	Lower Body	3 Mile Interval	Total Body/Core	Run 22 Miles

Week 27
Mon	Tue	Wed	Thur	Fri
Run 22 Miles	Lower Body	3 Mile Interval	Total Body/Core	Run 23 Miles

Week 30
Mon	Tue	Wed	Thur	Fri
Run 23 Miles	Lower Body	3 Mile Interval	Total Body/Core	Run 24 Miles

Week 31
Mon	Tue	Wed	Thur	Fri
Run 24 Miles	Lower Body	3 Mile Interval	Total Body/Core	Run 25 Miles

Week 32
Mon	Tue	Wed	Thur	Fri
Run 25 Miles	Lower Body	3 Mile Interval	Total Body/Core	Run 26 Miles

Lower Body Exercise

Since your legs bear much of the burden of carrying you through the run, it's important to give them some special attention. You need strong legs for a strong race.

Each day, choose up to five of these exercises. Either do timed sets or circuits. For timed sets, set a stop watch and do as many reps as you can finish in 90 seconds. When you've completed all the exercises, do them all again for 60 seconds, then do them all one more time for 30 seconds. Try to complete the series two to three times. For circuits, perform 15-20 repetitions of each exercise, depending on the weight you're using, and then do the circuit two to three more times. Choose from the exercises below:

Moves with weights

-Forward Lunges: Hold a barbell behind your shoulders and stand with your legs placed hip width apart. Step forward and lunge forward, with your knees bent 90 degrees angle abs tight and a straight back, drive through your heels and behind to get back to the start position. Repeat the move, switching legs.

-Rear Lunges: Holding a barbell behind your shoulders, with your feet placed hip distance apart, step back and lower into the lunge position. Drive through your heels and behind to go back to the start position. Repeat, switching legs.

-Squats: Hold a barbell behind your shoulders, with your legs slightly wider than hip width apart. Squat down as though you're sitting on a chair, keeping your abs pulled in and your back straight. Stand up to get back to the starting position. Repeat.

-Plie squats: Turn your toes out, with your feet spread wider than hip width. With your hands on your hips, and a dumbbell in each one, squat down, keeping your spine straight and abs and core tight. Stand up to get back to the starting position and repeat.

-Lateral Lunges: Stand with feet hip width apart, resting dumbbells on your hips. Step your foot out to the side and lower into a lunge position. Your knee shouldn't extend past your toes. Drive through the leg that's bent and go back to the start position. Repeat, switching sides.

-Calf Raises: Stand with your feet hip width apart and rest dumbbells on your hips. Drive through feet and bring your body up until you are on your tippy toes. Stay in this position for a single count and lower back to your feet. Repeat.

-Supinated Calf raises: With your feet slightly wider than hip width, a dumbbell in each hand, resting on your hips, turn your toes so that they are pointing inward, towards each other. (Pigeon-toed) Rise up on your tippy toes, for one count and lower down to your feet to get back starting position. Repeat.

-Pronated Calf Raises: With feet slightly wider than hip width and resting dumbbells on your hips, turn your feet out so your toes are pointing away from each other. Rise up to your tippy toes, hold for a single count and lower to your feet to get back to the starting position.

-Barbell Dead Lifts: Stand with feet hip width apart, with your shoulders back, and slightly arched. Lean forward from your hips and lower the barbell to the ground, or as close to it as you can.

Moves without weights

Every one of the moves above can be performed without weights, or you can choose from the moves below:

-Straight-leg Glute Extensions: Balance on your hands in knees, back straight, with weight evenly distributed. Kick your leg out behind you, with your knee straight. Hold it for a single count and get back to the starting position. Perform the move again, switching legs.

-Bent leg glute extensions: Balance on your hands and knees back straight, abs pulled into your spine weight evenly distributed. Lifting from your hip, bring your leg up behind you, with your knee bent 90 degrees. Hold for a single count and lower leg back to starting position. Repeat, switching legs.

-Hip Extension: Lie on your back, with abs pulled in. Lift your leg up until it is at a 90 degree angle to the floor, and lower back to the starting position without resting. Repeat, switching sides.

-Hip adduction: Lie on one side, with one leg bent over the other and one leg straight. Raise the straightened leg up as much as you can, hold for one count and lower it back down. Complete the reps and perform the moves on the other side.

-Hip abduction: Lie on your side, with your legs stacked on top of each other, placing on hand on the floor for support. Keep your top leg straight, lift it up until you can't lift anymore and lower back down to the starting position, without pausing. Complete the reps and perform the move on the opposite side.

-Wall sit: Stand with your back pressed against a wall and lower your body as though you're sitting in a chair. Hold for 30 seconds. Repeat as many times as you can.

-One leg balance/Squat: Balance on one leg as long as possible. If that's too easy, squat slightly. If it's still too easy, place any item on the floor, lower your body, on one leg, and touch the object, then raise up to standing.

-Stair running: Though this is usually considered a cardio workout, running up and down stairs does wonders for building strength in your lower body. If you have access to stairs, run up and down a flight as many times as you can.

Stability Ball

The stability ball is great for strengthening your legs, especially if your space is limited, or if you need to do moves that have little impact on your joints. Make sure your ball is the correct size. A customer service associate at a sporting goods store should be able to recommend the right size. Taller people need a larger sized stability ball than those on the short side.

As with the other exercises, you can perform these moves in a circuit or as timed sets. Some of the moves can be done with weights to make them more challenging.

-Ball squat on the wall: Squat down so your knees are 90 degrees, with the ball pressed against the wall and your back pressed on the ball. Place your hands behind your head or on your hips, and rise back up to the standing position for one rep. To perform this move with weights, follow the same steps, with your hands by your sides, a dumbbell in each one.

-One-legged ball squat on the wall: Stand on one leg, at 90 degrees, with your side against the stability ball, and the ball against the wall. Rise up to the standing position, and lower back down for one rep. Complete your set and repeat on opposite leg.

-One-legged ball squat without the wall: Ball behind you, your ankle placed on the top of the ball, step forward with your other leg. Bring your body down until your forward leg is bent at 90 degrees. Slowly rise until you're body is upright for one rep. Complete a set and switch sides.

-Ball toe-raise: Sit down, with your legs straight in front of you. Hold the ball between your ankles with you're your arms extended. Keeping your arms extended, flex your toes to bring the ball toward you. Squeeze for one count, then release for one rep. Make sure you are only using your calf muscles during this exercise.

-One-legged calf raise: Place the stability ball on a wall and lean with your chest pressed on the ball. Stand on one leg and lift your body so you are standing up on your toes, hold for a single count and lower back down for one rep. Complete your set and switch legs.

-Calf Raises: Perform the move the same as the one legged calf raises, but stand on both feet.

-Reverse Bridge: Lie down on your back with your feet on the ball, knees bent. Extend your legs and lift your back off of the floor. Slowly return back to the start position. That completes one rep. Make sure your back is straight throughout the exercise.

-Leg curls: Lie on your back and grip the ball under your knees using your knees and thighs to keep it up. Squeeze the ball and pull your feet toward your buttocks. Release and come back to start for one rep.

-Reverse leg curls: Lie face up with your feet on the ball. Bend your knees and use your feet to pull the ball toward you. Push the ball away from you and return to the start position to complete one rep.

-Hip abduction: Stand with your left side facing the wall. Use your left thigh, with your knee bent to hold the ball on the wall. Press your leg against the ball to squeeze it. Hold for one count and release. Complete your set and repeat on your right side.

-Hip adduction: Stand on your left leg and put your right foot on the ball, with your leg extended out to the side. Use your leg to take the ball back to you to complete one rep. Complete your set and repeat on left leg.

Total Body Moves

Your legs will get a serious workout during this training, and during the race itself, but that's not to say the rest of your body should be ignored. When running, your entire body is involved, so it should be involved during training.

We'll give you some moves that will give your entire body a major workout. Some of the moves might be more difficult than you anticipated, but don't quit. Quitters never win and winners never quit! Are we clear?

So gear up and get your work out on!

Circuit Training

Circuit training is a wonderful way to work multiple muscle groups at one time. They also save you time because of how many muscles you're working at once. Use the circuit below for one of your total-body days and you'll tighten up and build strength in your entire body. Perform 15-20 reps of each move, then rest for 60 seconds and repeat the sequence two to three times. You'll need a set of eight to fifteen pound dumbbells.

-Squat with overhead press: Stand with your feet together and your arms at shoulder height, weights by your ears. Lower into a squat as though you're sitting in a chair, and raise your arms to the parallel position at the same time. Return to the start position. That's one rep.

-Plank and reverse row: Get in the plank position, hands on weights, with your body in a straight line, your legs more than hip-width apart and arms directly underneath your shoulders. Keeping your abs pulled in and your core tight, lift your right elbow up and hold for one count. Lower the weight back to the floor and repeat on the left side.

-Side lunge: Stand with your feet and knees together, hands on hips. Step out to your right side, and bend your torso down from the waist. Don't round your spine and don't extend your right knee past your ankle. Step your right leg back in and get back to the start. Do the move again on your left side to complete one rep.

-Squat with arm raises: Stand with your legs wide and toes turned slightly out. Hold dumbbells with arms straight and palms down. Bend your knees to the point at which your thighs are parallel to the floor, while raising your arms up to shoulder height at the same time. Return to start to complete one rep.

-Side plank push-up: Sit on the floor, on your left side, with legs almost straight, and your right leg crossed over your left. Inhale, and lift your pelvis off the floor. To work your lats at the same time, pull your shoulder blade down to keep your shoulder away from your ear. Hold for five seconds to complete one rep. Complete your reps and switch sides.

-Rear Lunge and Bicep curl: Stand with back straight, feet hip width apart, with your arms down by your sides. Take a large step back and lower into a lunge, making sure your front knee doesn't extend passed the ankle. When you reach the bottom of the movement, perform a bicep curl. After you lower your arms, go back to start. Complete the move on the opposite side for one repetition.

-Russian twist: Sit down with your knees bent, and feet twenty-four inches from your buttocks. With your back straight, lean back a little. Make sure your spine is not rounded at any point while performing this move. Fully extend your arms out in front of you and place one hand over the other. Slowly twist to the right. Make sure the movement is from the rotating of your torso and not from the arm swing. Slowly rotate back to the center, then to the left for one rep.

-Ab Scissors: Lie flat on your back and place your hands by your sides or under your pelvis. Lift both of your legs toward the ceiling, keeping them straight. Slowly bring one leg down until it's about two inches from the floor, pause here, and release. Complete the move on your opposite side to complete one rep.

-Superman: Lie face down, with your neck in the neutral position, arms and legs extended. Lift your legs and arms off the floor at the same time, forming a "U" shape with your body. Hold for 30 seconds and repeat the move five times.

Kettlebells

These may very well be the Holy Grail of workout equipment. Kettlebells, which look sort of like a bowling ball that has a handle attached to it, do a number of things for your body. Since the weight of a kettlebell isn't evenly distributed, your stabilizer muscles work extra hard during every move you make with it. Your anaerobic systems is also working very hard when you use kettlebells because many of the moves bring your heart rate up really quickly. An hour long kettlebell workout can torch up to 1200 calories, perhaps the highest calorie burn known to man.

Perform the following circuit two to three times, doing five to ten reps of each movement. Increase your weight as you become more at ease with the moves.

-Two handed swing: Grip a kettlebell in one hand. Squat and release with one hand while grabbing it with the other. Continue passing the kettlebell from hand to hand for 15-30 reps. Start slowly when performing this move. You won't want your grip to fail and the kettlebell to go flying into your television or china hutch.

-Stand over the kettlebell with feet just a little wider than hip distance apart. Squat down and grip the kettlebell using an overhand grip. Extend your hips and knees to pull the kettlebell off the floor. Once it's off the floor, raise it over your shoulder, and jump upward, extending your entire body. Raise your shoulder and pull the kettlebell upward, allowing your elbow to bend slightly to the side. Now, drop under the kettlebell and rotate your arm underneath it. Catch it on the outside of your arm, with the kettlebell resting on your wrist. Move into a partial squat. Drive upward from your legs, driving the kettlebell up and over your head. Drop body down by bending your knees. Repeat the sequence.

-One handed swing: Follow the instructions of the two handed swing, but keep the kettlebell in the same and throughout the movement.

-Kettlebell windmill: Hold a kettlebell over head with your arm straight and near your ear. Push your hip out toward the arm that's holding the kettlebell and turn feet 45 degrees from the arm that's holding the kettlebell. Lower your body down until your non-working hand is touching the floor, or as close to the floor as you can reach. Repeat on the opposite side for one rep.

-Kettlebell Get-up/Turkish Get up: Lie on your back, holding a kettlebell overhead in your right arm aligned with your shoulder, fully extended. Bring your right leg in and pivot to your left. Roll onto your left triceps until your hand touches the floor. Drive forward, using your left and right leg. Bring in your left leg and bring your right leg forward, coming into a lunge position. Pause here, than stand up. If this move is too hard, begin with half-get ups. Lie on your back with the kettlebell in your right hand and your right knee bent. Rise up as though you are doing a sit up, keeping the kettlebell locked out over your head through the entire move. Lower back down for one rep. Complete reps and do them on the opposite side.

Please note: there are many, many more moves that can be performed with kettlebells. For even more, visit www.livestrong.com, www.bodybuilding.com or simply search for kettlebell exercises. If you like to get results fast, kettlebells are one very safe and effective way to do so.

Push-ups

An oldie but goodie, pushups are a time-honored exercise to increase strength in your chest, triceps and core. At the start or finish of every non-running workout, perform as many pushups as you can in two minutes. It doesn't sound like much, but it WORKS. In a few short weeks you'll notice that pushups are becoming easier, and your arms, shoulders and chest should tighten up. To vary the muscles you use, perform variations on your pushups. For example, do close-handed pushups one day, wide-grips on another, and staggered on another. This way you are targeting multiple muscle groups every time you do your pushups.

Sit ups

You want tight abdominal muscles when you run. Your abs support you and help keep your back straight, which goes far toward preventing injuries. The trick is to do sit ups the RIGHT way. Proper form is everything. Cross your arms over your chest and keep your chin tucked. Don't round your spine and control the motion during the entire exercise. Perform as many sit ups as you can in two minutes every day either before or after your workouts.

Don't forget oblique crunches, and reverse crunches, to make sure that most of the muscles in your abdominal region are being worked. When you start to feel a burn, do more sit ups. Your abs are big enough to work out every day. Unlike your other muscles they don't necessarily require as much rest between workouts, so don't be afraid to work them continually.

More About Your Core

Since your core is so vital to your run, and to fitness in general, we've include a chapter on how to keep it strong. Work your core on the days you do total body workouts and lower body workouts. While your abs are part of your core, there's much more to it than that. Your core is a huge series of muscles that work together to keep you upright and to move your arms and legs, so make sure you're taking care of it. A weak core leads to bad posture, which leads to bad running form, which leads to injuries. See why we don't like weakness?

Four for the Core

This four minute sequence does wonders for strengthening your entire core. Four minutes doesn't seem like much, but we promise it'll feel like you spent an hour on it.

-Minute one: Get in the plank position and hold it for one minute. Keep your back straight the entire time and your arms aligned with your shoulders.

-Minute two: Hold a left side plank for one minute. Keep your hips from dropping and keep your body straight.

-Minute three: Hold a right side plank for one minute, same as the left side, no dropping your hips.

-Minute four: Hold a traditional plank position for one minute.

Once you get used to this sequence, make it harder. While holding the plank position in minute one, punch your right arm in front of you, return it then punch out your left arm. Alternate your punches for the entire minute. While holding the plank for one minute, lift your right leg off the ground and hold for one count, then lift your left leg. Alternate your legs for the entire minute.

Another way to make planks harder: elevate your legs slightly while holding the position. Use a step, a curb, book, etc to lift your legs up.

Balancing act

Try performing any traditional dumbbell moves while off balance. Either stand on a Bosu ball or a rolled up towel. You will engage many muscles in your core while trying to maintain your balance, but you won't consciously work your core muscles.

Stability ball

The stability ball isn't just for your legs. Perform the moves below, as a circuit or as timed sets to build core strength and slim out your abs.

-Ball crunch: Lie down on the ball with it in your lower back. Tighten your abs and crunch up, with your hands crossed over your chest or your interlocked behind your head. Lower your torso back down. This completes one rep.

-Jack knife: Get in the push-up position, using the ball to elevate your legs. Draw your knees up to your chest to bring the ball toward you. Extend your legs out again. That's one rep.

-Ball reverse crunch: Grip the ball between your knees, while lying on your back. Lift your hips to bring the ball toward your chest. Bring your legs back down to complete one rep.

-Ball side crunch: Lie on one side with the ball under your rib cage. With your hands interlocked behind your head, crunch up, keeping your abs engaged. Lower your shoulders back down and repeat.

Interval Training

Interval training is important to building up your speed and cardio respiratory endurance. There are many types of interval training, but for the purpose of getting ready for a marathon, we'll focus on sprint intervals.

Because of the intensity of interval training, we don't advise doing more than three miles at a time, or up to 40 minutes of exercise. Alternate the workouts below on your short/fast run days.

High-Intensity Interval Sprint Workout:

-Do a five minute warm up

-Build up to a moderate pace, at an RPE (Rate of Perceived Exertion) of 5 for 5 Minutes

-Sprint as fast as you can for 30 seconds at an RPE of 9

-Bring your pace down to an RPE of 4-5 for 4.5 minutes

-Sprint for 30 seconds at an RPE of 9

-Bring your pace back to an RPE of 4-5 for 4.5 minutes

-Sprint for 30 seconds at an RPE of 9

-Cool down for 5 minutes.

Sixty One Twenties:

Do a five minute warm up, then perform 60/120 intervals. So what does this mean? Sprint for 60 seconds, with your RPE between 7-9, then walk or jog slowly for 120 seconds.

Repeat this sequence for 20 minutes, or do it ten to fifteen times.

Fartlek

Fartlek is Swedish for "speed play." It's similar to the HIIT workout above, but instead of timing your sprints, you'll use objects to determine how far you'll run. For instance, let's assume you're running on a sidewalk lined with streetlamps. Sprint from one street lamp to another, then jog from one to another. Keep this up for up to three miles. It's going to be hard, but don't quit. We don't like quitters!

Track Intervals

If you have access to a track, use it for interval runs if you need an easy way to measure your distance. Sprint on the straightway and walk or jog on the curves. Most tracks are a quarter of a mile, so it's easy to know how far you've run.

Treadmill Training

We don't like treadmill running. We train as we fight. You won't run your marathon on the treadmill, so you shouldn't train on it either. However, we know that inclement weather, or circumstances that prevent you from getting outside (children, visitors, someone's installing your cable, etc). We'd rather you use the treadmill than not run at all.

You can do a HIIT interval on the treadmill, or 60/120s. Be careful and don't set the speed higher than what you can manage. You still need to warm up and stretch in the same way you would if you were running outside.

Common Running Injuries

We have mentioned injury prevention ad nauseam, but it's only because we want you to finish your race. Being sidelined with a preventable injury sort of throws a monkey wrench in that. Since we care about you, we've included a chapter on injuries commonly associated with running, and how to prevent them.

So many people will tell you that running will cause bone and joint problems in the future. This is only true if you aren't doing the right thing now. Take care of yourself and follow our advice and you'll be able to run for the rest of your life, barring show stoppers such as a freak accident in the bathroom or other unanticipated catastrophe.

Achilles Tendonitis

Tendonitis in your Achilles is usually caused by overuse. The problem with this injury is that the Achilles doesn't get much blood, so it takes a long time to heal. You are especially susceptible to this injury during periods where you are trying to increase your speed or during hill runs. It doesn't mean you can't do them, but know your limits and start out slow. Signs of Achilles Tendonitis include pain and swelling in your ankles. If you experience these symptoms see a doctor to get a diagnosis and treatment.

Ignoring tendonitis can lead to the tendon snapping, which will likely require surgery to fix. Do you want to be laid up in the operating room on race day? We didn't think so.

Stress Reactions/Stress Fractures

Stress reactions, when left untreated can lead to the more severe injury, stress fractures. Fractures are caused by a one-time force that is stronger than the bone, which causes the bone to break. Unlike a fracture, a stress fracture is caused by a repetitive force that is more work than the bone can handle. When you put too much force on your bones, they can't heal before the next time they are impacted and a stress reaction or fracture occurs.

The most common sign of a stress fracture is a pain in the affected area that subsides over time. With continued impact placed on the joints, the pain will not subside, and can harm the effectiveness of your workout. If the pain persists even when you aren't working out, seek medical attention. Please be advised, a stress fracture IS a broken bone, so don't ignore it. Since they occur over time, it may be difficult to know when to see a doctor. When in doubt, ask the doctor.

Iliotibial (IT) Band Injury

IT injuries typically cause pain in the sides of your knees. This injury is caused when you don't ease yourself into speed runs. For example, when you sprint before a warm up, or when you try to run faster than what you body can handle. That's why we tell you to start slowly and why this program is so many weeks long. The injury can also be caused by wearing inappropriate running shoes, or pronation issues. Pronation means your feet turn in on impact, putting stress on your hips and knees.

Symptoms of IT band injury include lateral knee pain, which over time may radiate to your thighs. See a doctor if these symptoms occur. If you think you have a pronation problem, you may want to see an orthotic doctor who can help treat the issue with special footwear.

The best cure for this injury is rest and Non-steroidal anti-inflammatory drugs (NSAIDs).

Sprains

Strains are caused by a stretch or tear in the ligaments. This typically occurs when you trip and fall over stuff. To prevent it, watch where you're going, and keep up those balancing workouts so that you're less likely to fall.

To treat the injury, take it easy on running, but don't stop. Also, ice the affected area and take an NSAID.

Remember, only a doctor can correctly diagnose and treat any of these injuries, so if you are experiencing any sort of pain that you think is associated with running, don't attempt to fix it on your own. See a doctor who will help you establish a plan of care for the injury.

Avoiding Burn Out

We've provided a wide variety of workout options. However, if we haven't given you enough to keep boredom at bay, the following tips should be enough to keep it fun:

-Find a "battle buddy." Recruit one of your friends to join you in training. Just don't meet up for a high calorie brunch after training.

-Change your scenery. Don't use the same run route every day. When you run past the same buildings and land marks every day, you may get bored. To avoid this, map out several routes to choose from on your run days. Pick your route the night prior to the run.

-Work out to a beat. Create several playlists of the songs that get you pumped up and play them during your workout. Music tends to make you work out harder and makes the time pass faster.

-Read health magazines. If you don't like the workouts we've created, you can customize our program with plans you find in magazines. You can also find more recipes and helpful tips.

-Reward yourself. Set milestones for yourself during training and do something nice for yourself (that doesn't involve fatty cakes) every time you reach a milestone.

Women, feel free to get a manicure or facial. Men, treat yourself to a sporting event or a (light) beer.

-Take up sports. Once in a while, rather than doing strength training, get some friends together for a competition. You still want to get a good workout, so choose high energy sports such as football, soccer, basketball, volleyball or street hockey.

-Take a class. If sports aren't your thing, look into taking an aerobics class at your gym on some days, to break up your routine. Try spinning, step aerobics, or Zumba!

Don't get bored, whatever you do. Boredom will cause your performance to plummet and kill your motivation. Without motivation you'll never go the distance.

Crossing The Finish Line

We are confident that following this plan will bring you to the finish line on race day. We know you'll have "off" days, but don't get discouraged. Keep up with it and you won't regret it!

Resource Section

RunnersDepot.org – Your full line of gear for all things running.

You can find every piece of equipment mentioned in this book at RunnersDepot.org

Smoothies For Runners – Excellent book by CJ Hitz for runners and smoothie lovers alike!

(http://www.runnersdepot.org/smoothies.htm)

Made in the USA
San Bernardino, CA
08 November 2012